Patients Knowledge Assessment on Vitamin K Antagonist

First Printing: 2020

ISBN: 978-1-71651-276-6

Affiliation of Author

Vaishnavi Ananda Padmanabhan,
Guru Nanak Institutions Technical Campus-School of Pharmacy,
Ibarhimpatnam, Ranga Reddy District, Hyderabad,
Telangana, India- 501506.

Sahithi Reddy Kondapalli
Guru Nanak Institutions Technical Campus-School of Pharmacy,
Ibarhimpatnam, Ranga Reddy District, Hyderabad,
Telangana, India- 501506.

Sagar Pamu
Guru Nanak Institutions Technical Campus-School of Pharmacy,
Ibarhimpatnam, Ranga Reddy District, Hyderabad,
Telangana, India- 501506.

www.lulu.com
Lulu Press, Inc
627 Davis Drive, Suite 300, Morrisville, NC 27560.

Patients Knowledge Assesment on Vitamin K Antagonist

Author

Vaishnavi Ananda Padmanabhan

Sahithi Reddy Kondapalli

Sagar Pamu

Editor

Sagar Pamu

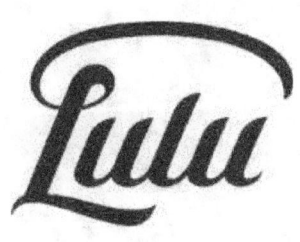

2019

About Author

Vaishnavi Ananda Padmanabhan, pursued Pharm.D at Guru Nanak Institutions Technical Campus- School of Pharmacy (GNITC-SOP). She attended and presented in various conferences and seminars on different topics related to clinical pharmacy. She has an experience of patient counselling during medical camps and she achieved top score during academics.

Sahithi Reddy Kondapalli, pursued Pharm.D at GNITC-SOP. She has skills in ADR detection & prescription analysis. She also attended and presented in various conferences & seminars. She also has an experience of patient counseling during medical camps. She has an excellent experience in dealing patients during hospital visit.

Sagar Pamu, Pharm.D, is an Assistant Professor in GNITC-SOP. He filed one patent, authored 19 articles in international & national journals and 20 books. He also participated and presented in various national conferences and seminars.

Acknowledgement

At the very outset, we thank God, the Almighty for showering his blessings and being a source of guidance and wisdom throughout the study without which no human achievement is possible.

*We are indebted to our beloved **Parents** without whose encouragement and help our professional career would never see the light of the day.*

As we walk along the path of life, we have the pleasure of meeting people who search our life in such a way that it never is the same gain...it may be small thoughtful things they do, a smile, a helping hand, a word of encouragement or just by mere presence they make our life worth living.

Accomplishing this project has been a great learning and very fulfilling experience. There have been many people who have come along side and helped in conceiving, designing, and executing this project. I would like to place a record and my sincere appreciation for their contribution.

"Words cannot be said nor written for obligation and indebtedness"

*We take immense pleasure in thanking my research guide **Dr. Praneeth Polamuri, MD, DM, Department of cardiology, Care Hospitals** for his rejuvenating inspiration, kind co-operation, valuable guidance, suggestions and encouragement throughout the progress of this work which helped me to complete every aspect of this project work and for his generous offer to use the available data on Primary PCI patients.*

We wish to extend my sincere thanks to my co-guides **Dr. Praveen, MD, DM, Dr. Rahul Agarwal, Intensive Cardiologist**, *for their kind co-operation, valuable guidance, suggestions and encouragement, encouragement at every step, and continuous assistance right from conceptualization of the project work for the preparation of this thesis.*

We heartily thank **Mrs. T. Lakshmi, HOD of Pharm- D,** *my research guide for her tolerance, keen interest, valuable guidance, logical thoughts, kind co-operation, constructive criticism, and encouragement in every step, and continuous assistance right from conceptualization of the project work to the preparation of this thesis and suggestions which helped me to complete every aspect of this project work.*

Just as a music conductor is important for an orchestra, the Principal of a college is pivotal. My principal, teacher **Dr. T. Rama Rao, Associate Director and Principal,** *never went back in taking personal interest, providing constant encouragement and valuable advice. I am deeply thankful for facilitating the project and creating a conductive environment for completing the project.*

We immensely thankful to **Dr. B Soma Raju, Chairman and Managing Director, Care Hospitals**, *for his rejuvenating inspiration, valuable suggestions and encouragement given to me during the project work.*

We would like to express my deep sense of gratitude to **Dr. N Krishna Reddy, Vice Chairman,** *for his guidance, valuable suggestions and affection during my course.*

We immensely thankful to **Dr. Raghava Raju, Medical Director**, *for his kind co-operation, inspiring guidance, supervision and help in completing this work.*

*We would like to express my sincere gratitude and feels immense pleasure in thanking to **Dr. Anuj Kapadiya, MD, DM, Director of Cath Lab services**, for his guidance during the term of my project. Without his valuable assistance, this work would not have been completed.*

*We profusely thank **Dr. Riyaz Khan, Facility chief operating officer,** for the infrastructure and all other essential facilities and encouragement given to us during the project work.*

*We take the privilege to express my heart full gratitude to **Dr. Gopi Krishna, Medical Superintendent, Dr. S. Naga Satish Kumar, Associate Medical Superintendent and Dr. Harish Jawalkar, Associate Medical Superintendent** for their co-operation, affection, encouragement and moral support throughout our project.*

*We wish to extend my sincere thanks to **Dr. Naresh, DNB Cardiologist** for encouragement, timely help in my project work and support.*

*We express my sincere thanks to **Mr. Venkatesh, Clinical Pharmacist and Research Coordinate, and Mr. Vidya Sagar, Clinical Pharmacist** for their cooperation and help in completing this work.*

*It is my privilege to express thanks to **Dr. J. N. Narendra Sharath Chandra** for encouragement and moral support throughout the project.*

*Our sincere thanks to **Mr. Sudheer** for his help and guidance in performing statistics of the study.*

*We would be failing in my duty if I don't acknowledge the help of **Authors** of journals and books, the sentinels of my project work.*

Our sincere thanks to senior's and my entire batch mates, for all the love, support they have given throughout my **Pharm D** *and letting me be me and realize my potential.*

Finally, yet importantly, we thank all the **Patients** *who participated in the study without whom the study would not be possible.*

Thanks again……

By,

Vaishnavi Ananda Padmanabhan,
Sahithi Reddy Kondapalli.

Dedication

Dedicated to my beloved Parents, Teachers and
Friends

Thank you. Without your support and patience, I
would have never achieved my dream

Table of Contents

List of Tables

List of Figures

Chapter-I

Introduction

Vitamin K Antagonists

Vitamin K is essential for the synthesis of multiple factors in the coagulation cascade: Factors II (prothrombin), VII, IX and X, as well as protein C and protein S. Vitamin K Antagonists (VKA) have been used as anticoagulants for over 50 years. Warfarin, a synthetic derivative of coumarin, is the most commonly used VKA, although other coumarin derivatives (phenprocoumon and acenocoumarol) are also used

Limitations of Vitamin K Antagonists

Limitations of VKAs include:

o Narrow therapeutic window

o Interactions with drugs and food (e.g. foods rich in vitamin K)

o Delayed onset and offset of anticoagulant effect (this is a particular limitation for prevention of venous thromboembolism, in which the duration of therapy is relatively short).

o Need for frequent coagulation monitoring and dosage adjustments.

o Variable dose-response between individuals

Monitoring Vitamin K Antagonists

Because of the variability in the dose-response with VKA medications, monitoring the degree of anticoagulation is imperative. The prothrombin time (PT) is sensitive to changes in prothrombin, Factor VII, Factor IX and Factor X. Because of variability in the test reagent, thromboplastin, haematology laboratories now use an international INR for the measurement of PT prolongation. The INR provides a standardized measure of the VKA anticoagulant effect and should be kept within a narrow range to control the intensity of anticoagulation in patients taking VKAs. For most conditions for which VKAs are prescribed, the recommended therapeutic INR range is 2.0–3.0

- o As the INR increases, the risk of bleeding increases, doubling with each one-point increase in INR
- o A patient's INR should be monitored frequently when:
- o A VKA is started
- o The dose is changed
- o There are changes in diet or medications known to interact with VKAs

Once a stable dose that produces a therapeutic INR level is reached, the test ideally should be repeated every 4 weeks. Polymorphisms in the genes for cytochrome P450 2C9 (which is responsible for the metabolic clearance of warfarin) and vitamin K epoxide reductase (which recycles vitamin K) affect the pharmacodynamics of warfarin, contributing to a variable dose-response between individuals [3]. Research is currently in progress on the clinical utility of genetic polymorphism testing to guide VKA dosing

Uses of oral VKA

Oral fat-soluble vitamin antagonist medicine square measure was wont to forestall and treat thrombosis and pulmonic clot and to forestall blood vessel thromboembolism in patients with arrhythmia or cardiac disease, including mechanical heart valves.

Examples :

- Warfarin (Coumadin)
- Coumatetralyl.
- Phenprocoumon.
- Acitrom (Acenocoumarol).
- Dicoumarol.
- Tioclomarol.
- Brodifacoum.

The story of warfarin leads us from a mysterious haemorrhagic disease of cattle to the development of a rat poison which became one of the most commonly prescribed drugs in history. Many people were involved in the story and we owe them all a debt of gratitude.

The Discovery of Warfarin

The sweet clover problem: Warfarin is the most widely used anticoagulant in the world. In the UK it is estimated that at least 1% of the population and 8% of the over-80s are taking it regularly (Pirmohamed, 2006). The fascinating story of its discovery begins on the prairies of Canada and the Northern Plains of America in the 1920s.

Previously healthy cattle in these areas began dying of internal bleeding with no obvious precipitating cause. Given that livestock was one of the most important industries in these areas and because most North Americans were already severely economically wounded by The Great Depression, this was a devastating blow for the farmers' livelihoods. As there was an apparent lack of a recognisable pathogenic organism or nutritional deficiency responsible for the hemorrhage, the diet of the livestock was questioned. The cattle and sheep had grazed on sweet clover hay (*Melilotusalba* and *Melilotusofficinalis*) and the incidence of bleeding occurred most frequently when the climate, and therefore the hay, in these areas were damp. Such damp hay became infected by moulds such as *Penicilliumnigricans* and *Penicilliumjensi* which appeared to be integral in the disease process occurring in the cattle (Schofield, 1924; Roderick, 1929, 1931). As Duxbury and Poller point out in their review article on warfarin, such hay would normally have been discarded if it spoiled in storage but in the financial hardship of the 1920s few farmers could afford to buy supplementary fodder for their cattle and thus the mouldy hay was used to feed them (Duxbury &Poller, 2001). The resultant hemorrhagic disease, which became known as 'sweet clover disease', became manifest within 15 d of ingestion and killed the animal within 30–50 d (Duxbury &Poller, 2001). Schofield and Roderick, two local veterinary surgeons, had demonstrated sweet clover disease to be potentially reversible if the offending mouldy hay was removed, or if fresh blood was transfused into the bleeding animals (Schofield, 1924; Roderick, 1929). The recommendations to local farmers were that they should avoid feeding their cattle with the mouldy sweet clover hay. Roderick showed that the acquired coagulation disorder was caused by what he called a 'plasma prothrombin defect' (Roderick, 1929).

Isolation of the oral anticoagulant

Ten years after the original outbreak of sweet clover disease, a young Wisconsin farmer, Ed Carlson, was at his wits' end from losing so many of his prized cows and bulls from internal bleeding. Like so many local farmers he had no faith in the theory of sweet clover disease. After all, they had fed the cows with the hay for generations and to no ill effect. One winter's day he travelled 200 miles in a blizzard, with a dead cow in the back of his truck, to the local agricultural experimental station where investigators Karl Link and his senior student Wilhelm Schoeffel was working. As the story goes, Carlson entered Link's office (the only one he found open in the building) carrying milk can of unclotted blood. Although sympathetic, all that Link could recommend was the avoidance of the mouldy hay and the possibility of a transfusion of blood, as Schofield and Roderick had demonstrated some years previously. IN (fig 1)Karl Link had only become interested in the sweet clover problem a month earlier. Nonetheless, it would appear that Carlson had indeed come to the right place. Schofield experimented with the blood that evening and, as Duxbury and Poller comment, 'The can of uncoagulated blood lying on the floor of Link's laboratory was to change the course of history, and little did Link know what the long-term implications would be' (**Duxbury &Poller, 2001**). Although the cause of the haemorrhagic malady had been found, in the sweet clover, the actual active compound had yet to be identified or even isolated. Link and colleagues got to work on finding the active substance from the spoiled hay.

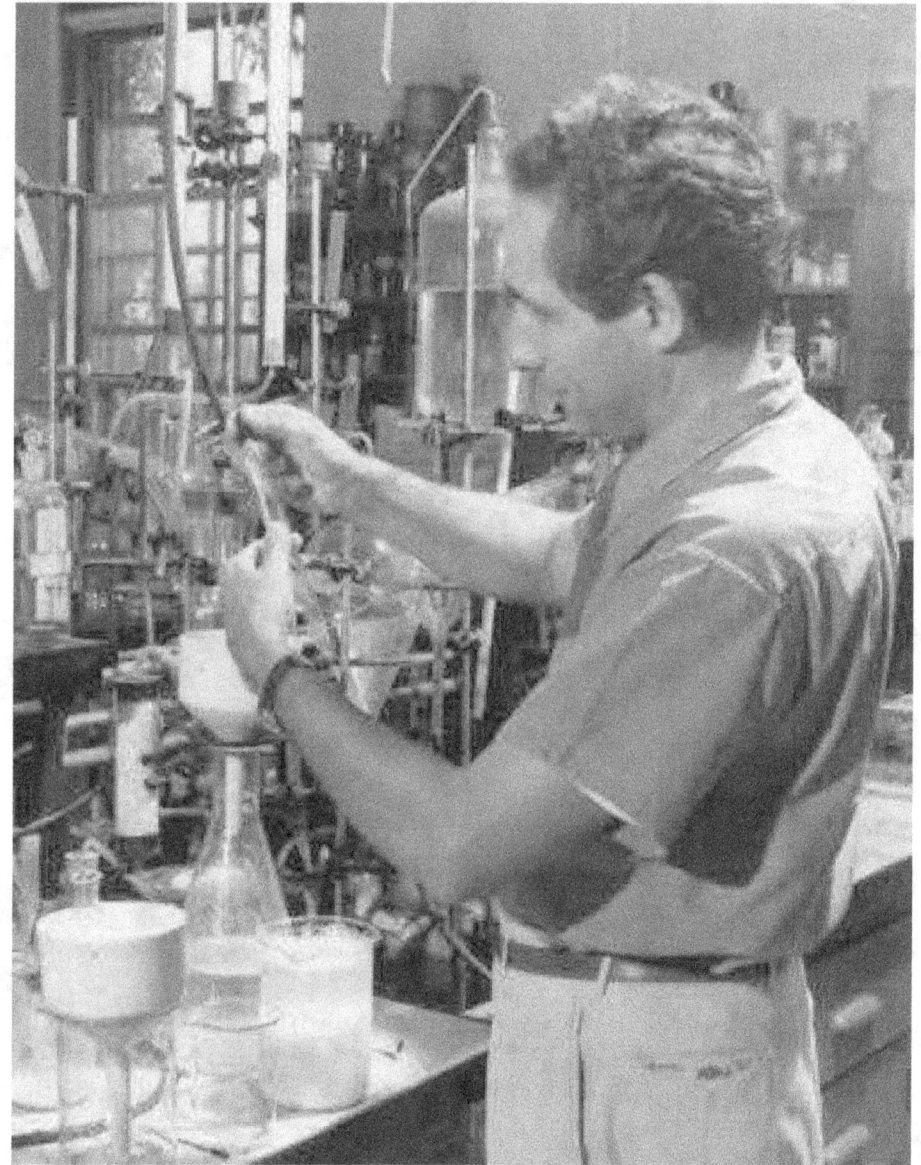

Fig 1: Karl Link in his laboratory (courtesy of University of Wisconsin)

A new in vitro clotting assay using plasma from rabbits was developed to guide chemical fractionation of compounds found in the hay. After some 6 years of intensive work, Link's laboratory was finally able to crystallise the substance. It proved to be 3,3¢-methylene-bis[4-

hydroxycoumarin] (Camp-ballet al, 1940, 1941; Campbell & Link, 1941; Stahmannet al,1941). They found that that natural coumarin became oxidised in mouldy hay, to form the substance that would become better known as dicoumarol. Large scale isolation of dicoumarol was accomplished by graduate student Mark Stahmann who went on to become a professor of the biochemistry department at Wisconsin (Last, 2002). The work was funded by the Wisconsin Alumni Research Foundation (WARF), and patent rights for dicoumarol were given to WARF in 1941.

From test tube to rat poison in 1945, whilst recovering in a sanatorium from 'wet pleurisy', Link got the idea of using a coumarin derivative as a rodenticide, the rodents dying of internal haemorrhage. He reviewed all the bioassay data to select the best variations of dicoumarol to create what he called 'better mousetraps'. He thought dicoumarol a poor rodenticide because it acted too slowly (Last, 2002). Link and colleagues, still funded by WARF began working on several variations of the naturally occurring coumarin. Number 42 of a list of 150 appeared to be particularly active; warfarin (named after the authority the financial muscle that funded the research) was born as shown in (figure2). It was promoted in 1948 as a rodenticide.

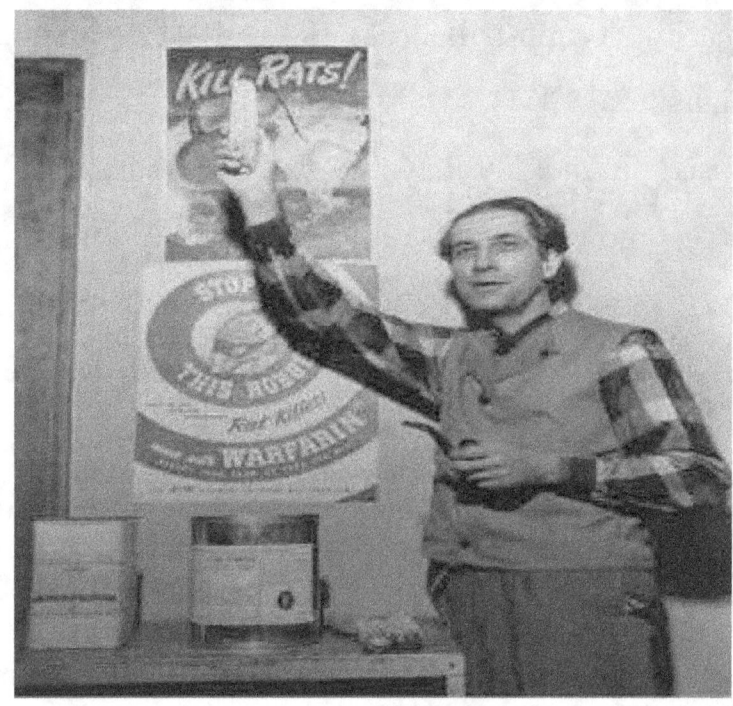

Fig 2: Karl Link promoting warfarin as a rodenticide (courtesy of the University of Wisconsin)

From Rat Poison to Clinical Application

After its success as a rodenticide, the transition of Coumadin to the clinical application was created beneath the name 'Coumadin'.Other anticoagulants were available; however, of those anticoagulant medications needed epithelial duct administration and dicoumarol had an extended latent amount before the onset of therapeutic impact. The principal advantages of warfarin were its high water solubility and high oral bioavailability (Last, 2002). It was more potent than dicoumarol but retained the ability to have its effect reversed by vitamin K (Overman al, 1942).In 1955, Warfarin was given to President Dwight Eisenhower following a myocardial infarction As Duxbury and Poller point out; 'What was good for a war hero and thePresident of the United States must be good for all, despite being a rat poison!' (Duxbury &Poller, 2001). A major problem in the widespread clinical application of warfarin proved to be the laboratory method used for dosage control; the prothrombin time (PT). In the 1950s, commercial sources of thromboplastin became available but they varied markedly in their responsiveness to the defect induced by vitamin K antagonists. As a result, the Pt varied greatly betting on the factor III used. Expressing the results as a prothrombin ratio (PTR) did not solve the problem. If less with responsive commercial thromboplastins were used larger doses were given to meet the target PTR. This led to overdosage and widespread reports of bleeding. In the united kingdom, a lot of sensitive factor III was used then within the USA and it became clear that the UK had fewer haemorrhage complications. It was later accomplished that if samples area unit taken from patients on vitamin K antagonists and also the PTs or PTRs obtained with 2 completely different thromboplastins planned against one another in a log-log plot the points lay on a straight line. Based on this fact the World Health Organisation (WHO) in 1982 adopted a model to convert the PTR obtained with any reagent to an international normalised ratio (INR) that is the PTR that would have been obtained if an International Reference Preparation (IRP) had been used (Kirkwood, 1983; WHO Expert Committee on Biological Standardization, 1983). If the PTRs using the IRP are plotted on the y-axis and the PTRs using the local laboratory reagent on the X-axis the slope of the line is known as the International Sensitivity Index (ISI). The INR is then the PTR found in the local laboratory raised to the power of the ISI. This system standardised anticoagulant control worldwide.

Moving into the modern era of clinical trials

The first randomised trial of these anticoagulants was performed in 1960 (Barritt& Jordan, 1960). Patients with pulmonary embolism were randomised to anticoagulation with heparin and nicoumalone or to no anticoagulation. Of the 16 patients randomised to anticoagulation, none died from a pulmonary embolism and there were no non-fatal recurrences. Of the 19 patients randomised to no treatment, five died from a pulmonary embolism and there were also five non-fatal recurrences. The importance of the initial treatment with heparin was confirmed much more recently when heparin plus acenocoumarol was compared with acenocoumarol alone for the initial treatment of proximal deep vein thrombosis (Brandjes et al, 1992). In the 60 patients treated with heparin and acenocoumarol, there were no extensions of the thrombus and there were two pulmonary emboli and two recurrences. In the 60 patients treated with acenocoumarol alone, there were two extensions of the thrombus, two pulmonary emboli and eight recurrences. The importance of heparin was also illustrated by studies that looked at the adequacy of the dose (Hull et al, 1986; Raschke et al, 1993). Hull et al (1986) compared subcutaneous and intravenous heparin for the treatment of proximal DVT. It was noticed that irrespective of the mode of delivery, inadequate heparinisation in the first 24 h resulted in a 25% recurrence rate whilst it was only 1Æ6% in those adequately anticoagulated. Raschke et al (1993) compared two intravenous heparin regimens []. The fixed-dose regimen resulted in inadequate anticoagulation in 68% at 6 h and 23% at 24 h, the figures for the weight-based regimen were 14 and 3% respectively.

The risk of recurrent thromboembolism was fivefold greater in the former group. From these studies, it seemed that an inadequate activated partial thromboplastin time response to unfractionated heparin in the first 24 h coagulant control worldwide increased the risk of recurrence. However, a meta-analysis has suggested that this does not seem to be critical if the starting rate is at least 1250 U/h (Anand et al, 1996). The dosing of warfarin was also controversial (see above). Was dosing in the UK too low, increasing the incidence of thrombosis, or was the dosing in the USA excessive, leading to unacceptable bleeding risks? The matter was resolved in a randomised trial in which patients with venous thrombo-embolism were assigned to a target PTR of 2Æ0–3Æ0 using either the British thromboplastin (supplied by Dr Leon Poller) or the less sensitive thromboplastin used at McMaster Hospital. The incidence of recurrent thrombosis was 2% in both groups but bleeding rates were five times higher if the North Americanthromboplastin was used (22% vs. 4%) (Hullet al, 1982). As the British reagent had an ISI of 1Æ0 this lent to the widespread adoption of an INR target of 2Æ0–3Æ0. Low molecular weight heparins have now largely replaced unfractionated heparin. The key reason is that they produce a much more predictable anticoagulant response. This combined with the fact that they have very high bioavailability after subcutaneous injection means that the dose can be calculated by body weight and be given subcutaneously without any monitoring or dose adjustment. They are at least as effective and at least as safe as unfractionated heparin even when given once a day and this made out-patient treatment possible(Koopman et al, 1996; Levine et al, 1996). We now await the results of phase III clinical trial of direct oral thrombin inhibitors and direct oral anti-factor Xa inhibitors. This drug will surely be available in the next few years. Will, they are suitable for all patients and for all indications (no trials are taking place in patients with prosthetic heart valves)? We are left to speculate whether heparin and warfarin will still be used100 years after their discover

Mechanism of Action

Warfarin acts by inhibiting the synthesis of vitamin k dependent clotting factors, which include Factors II, VII, IX, and X.Vitamin K is an essential cofactor for the post ribosomal synthesis of the vitamin K-dependent clotting factors. Vitamin K promotes the biosynthesis of γ-carboxyglutamic acid residues in the proteins that are essential for biological activity. Warfarin interferes with clotting factor synthesis by inhibition of the C1 subunit of vitamin K epoxide reductase (VKORC1) enzyme complex, thereby reducing the regeneration of vitamin K_1 epoxide. [1][4]

Indications

➢ Prophylaxis and treatment of venous thrombosis, pulmonary embolism (PE).

- Prophylaxis and treatment of thromboembolic complications associated with atrial fibrillation (AF) and/or cardiac valve replacement (metallic and non-metallic).

- Reduction in the risk of death, recurrent myocardial infarction (MI), and thromboembolic events such as stroke or systemic embolization after myocardial infarction. [1][4][5][8]

Contraindication

- Hemorrhagic tendencies or blood dyscrasias

- Recent or contemplated surgery of the central nervous system or eye, or traumatic surgery resulting in large open surfaces

- Bleeding tendencies associated with Active ulceration or over bleeding of the gastrointestinal, genitourinary, or respiratory tract

- Central nervous system haemorrhage

- Cerebral aneurysms, dissecting aorta

- Pericarditis and pericardial effusions

- Bacterial endocarditis

- In women who are pregnant except in pregnant women with mechanical heart valves, who are at high risk of thromboembolism.

- Exposure while pregnancy causes an evident pattern of major congenital malformations (warfarin embryopathy and fetotoxicity), fatal fetal haemorrhage, and an increased risk of spontaneous abortion and fetal mortality. Threatened abortion, eclampsia, and pre-eclampsia. [1][4][5][8].

Adverse Drug Reactions

The common ADRs as per previous studies are tissue Necrosis, Calciphylaxis, Acute Kidney Injury, Systemic Atheroemboli and Cholesterol Microemboli, Limb Ischemia, Necrosis, and Gangrene Patients with HIT and HITTS [1][4][5]

Immune System Disorders

Hypersensitivity / Allergic Reactions (including urticaria and anaphylactic reactions).

Vascular Disorders – Vacuities, Cholestatic Hepatitis has been associated with concomitant administration of warfarin and ticlopidine.

Gastrointestinal Disorders - Nausea, Vomiting, Diarrhoea, Taste perversion, Abdominal.

Hepatobiliary Disorders - Hepatitis, elevated liver enzymes. pain, flatulence, bloating.

Skin Disorders- Rash, Dermatitis (including bullous eruptions alopecia.

Respiratory Disorders - Tracheal or Tracheobronchial Calcification.

General Disorders – Chills. [1][4][5]

Dosage –

- Individualized Dosing by repeated measurement of prothrombin time
- The dosage and administration of warfarin must be individualized for each patient according to the patient's INR response to the drug.
- Adjust the dose based on the patient's INR and the condition being treated

- The optimum ratio of pt during treatment with the oral anticoagulant to the normal value has been defined for various indications.

A standardized system called the international normalized ratio (INR) based on the use of human brain has been developed by WHO and adopted in all countries

Target (INR) for Various Indications

The target INR for each indication is given in table no: 1

Table No. 1: Target INR for each Indication

Indications	INR
Prophylaxis of deep vein thrombosis and a similar indication	2-2.5
Treatment of deep vein thrombosis-pulmonary embolism, toes, hip surgery	2-3
Recurrent thromboembolism, arterial disease (mi), prosthetic heart valves	3-3.5

Monitoring Warfarin

INR test meters may be prescribed to patients for use in the home, and they may also be used by health care providers. However, India is not so famous with this practice and is also not economical for the Indian population. How often an INR is monitored and the results a patient should expect, will be based on the advice from the physician.

An INR target range is typically between 2.0 and 3.0 for basic blood-thinning, anyhow the range may vary based on a patient's conditions.medication dose is changed according to INR Patients should work with their physician for achieving and maintaining a target INR[6][8][9].

Pharmacokinetics and Pharmacodynamics

Warfarin is a racemic mixture of a right-handed and a left-handed stereoisomer, designated R and S. This racemic mixture has a half-life of approximately 36 to 42 hours. The S-isomer is five times more potent as a vitamin K antagonist than the R-isomer.9 Absorption of warfarin is rapid and complete. It is highly protein-bound (> 98%), primarily to albumin. Only the free drug is pharmacologically active.10 If the serum albumin level is low (such as in the nephrotic syndrome), the free fraction of warfarin is increased, but so is its plasma clearance.11 Therefore, such conditions are not likely to lead to significant changes in the INR. The hepatic metabolism of the two isomers differs, with clinically significant implications for drug interactions. The S-isomer is primarily metabolized by cytochrome P450 2C9 (and to a lesser degree by P450 3A4) and is eliminated in the bile. The R-isomer, in contrast, is primarily metabolized by cytochrome P450 1A2 and P450 3A4 and is excreted in the urine as inactive metabolites. Since the S-isomer is much more potent than the R-isomer, medications that inhibit or induce the P450 2C9 pathway lead to the most significant drug interactions. Most drug interactions that affect the R-isomer are not significant.

Starting Warfarin

Warfarin is commonly used to decrease the risk of systemic arterial thromboembolism (eg, Warfarin can paradoxically exert a procoagulant response by interfering with proteins C and S WARFARIN DOSING JAFFER AND BRAGG What to tell a patient taking warfarin Indicate the reason for starting warfarin and how it relates to clot formation Review the trade name and generic name of the drug and discuss how warfarin works Discuss the potential duration of therapy Explain the need for frequent INR testing and the target INR appropriate for the patient's treatment Describe the common signs and symptoms of bleeding Describe the common signs and symptoms of a thrombotic event Outline precautionary measures to decrease trauma or bleeding Discuss the influence of dietary vitamin K Discuss potential drug interactions (prescription, over-the-counter, herbal) Discuss the need to avoid or limit alcohol consumption Explain need for birth control measures for women of childbearing age Stress the importance of notifying all their health care providers (physicians, dentists, etc) that they are taking warfarin Ask patient to notify the anticoagulation provider when dental, surgical, or invasive procedures and hospitalization are scheduled or occur unexpectedly Ask patient to notify anticoagulation provider of any change in warfarin tablet color, shape, or markings Specify when to take warfarin and what to do if they miss a dose Instruct patient about the importance of carrying identification in patients with atrial fibrillation or flutter or prosthetic valves. It is also used to prevent recurrent venous thromboembolism in patients with deep vein thrombosis or pulmonary embolism. Less commonly, it is used for secondary prevention after myocardial infarction. When starting anticoagulation therapy, it is always important to review the risks and benefits with the patient. The decision should incorporate the patient's medical, social, dietary, and medication history, level of education and understanding, health beliefs, and adherence to prior therapy. [12]

Subsequently, the patient should be thoroughly educated about warfarin"What you need to know about your warfarin therapy," pon initiation of therapy and periodically thereafter. A system, either written or electronic, should be developed for documenting and recording test results, patient encounters, and return visits. Nomograms and computer programs are available to guide dosing.

Importance of the INR

The INR was developed in 1982 by the World Health Organization's Expert Committee on Biologic Standardization in response to variations in thromboplastin sensitivity and different ways of reporting the prothrombin time across the world.8 Inappropriate management can lead to subtherapeutic or supratherapeutic INR values, increasing the risk of acute or recurrent thromboembolic episodes or bleeding episodes, respectively. For most indications, the therapeutic INR range is 2.0 to 3.0. Exceptions are when warfarin is used for secondary prevention after myocardial infarction or for patients with high-risk mechanical prosthetic heart valves, in which case the range is 2.5 to 3.5.

Maintenance Therapy

Once a patient makes the transition from the initial dosing phase to the maintenance phase, more consideration to the multiple factors that may affect the INR should be given when interpreting low or high INR values. The key is to individualize the dosage according to these factors and the target INR range. The ideal regimen should provide the same dose every day, but this is not always possible. Warfarin comes in many tablet strengths: 1, 2, 2.5, 3, 4, 5, 6, 7.5, and 10 mg. Still, for some patients, a given tablet strength might not be enough while the next higher tablet strength may be too much. In this situation, one needs to give different doses on different days of the week. It is better if the doses are similar rather than greatly different. For example, if a patient were taking warfarin 2 mg daily except 4 mg on Monday and Friday using 2-mg tablets, it would be reasonable to change the dosage to 3 mg daily except 2 mg on Monday, Wednesday, and Friday if the INR tended to fluctuate regularly. The patient would still receive 18 mg/week, but with less variability in the day-to-day dose. This type of regimen may not work for every patient, as it could be confusing or the patient may have difficulty splitting tablets. Nevertheless, the point is that the warfarin dosage needs to be individualized. In most cases, alternating doses (eg, 2.5 mg alternating with 5 mg) or repeating doses (eg, 2.5 mg, then 2.5 mg, then 5 mg) should be avoided, as they provide different total weekly doses of warfarin. Before changing the dosage

Before adjusting the dosage of warfarin, one should evaluate previous warfarin doses, previous rapid anticoagulant effect does not equal an antithrombotic effect WARFARIN DOSING JAFFER AND BRAGG ous INR results, and whether anything else in the patient's condition or regimen has changed. Patients should be asked about

• Adherence. Did they miss any doses?

• Changes in other medications. Asking if any medication changes have occurred since the last INR may be too vague—it may be necessary to inquire more specifically: Did you start any prescription drugs, over-the-counter drugs, or herbal or natural remedies since your last visit? Did you stop any of these? Did the dosage of any of these changes? Any of these can alter warfarin's action.

• Current vitamin K consumption, including foods, vitamins, and supplements.

• Concomitant illnesses.

Patients with medical conditions that may affect warfarin such as congestive heart failure or thyroid dysfunction should be asked about disease-specific symptoms or medication changes. Although every instance doesn't need to ask about recent illness, remember that illness can affect the INR in several ways. Fever, vomiting, or diarrhoea can affect INR. Ill patients may reduce their intake of vitamin K. Antibiotics may alter the response to warfarin

Causes of High or Low INRs

Many things can cause the INR to become high or low. This is not intended to be an exhaustive review of all such causes but to provide a concise overview. Since there are multiple causes to consider, you should not assume that one patient's response to a particular effect will hold for all subsequent patients. This highlights the need for a thorough assessment of any abnormal INR value and an individualized approach to dosage adjustments and follow-up monitoring of the INR.

Drug Interactions:

Of the many causes of high or low INR values, the most common that are likely to lead to significant changes in the INR and increase the propensity for bleeding or clotting are drug interactions. Drug interactions with warfarin can be defined as either pharmacokinetic or pharmacodynamic. Pharmacokinetic interactions involve alterations in the absorption, protein binding, and hepatic metabolism of warfarin. Conversely, pharmacodynamic interactions affect the tendency for bleeding or clotting through either antiplatelet effects or increases or decreases in vitamin K catabolism. Pharmacokinetic interactions. Few medications affect the absorption of warfarin. The most widely cited example is cholestyramine, and this interaction may be minimized or avoided by separating the doses of warfarin and cholestyramine by 2 to 6 hours. Interactions involving protein binding displacement are few and usually of minimal significance since a compensatory increase in plasma clearance of warfarin occurs with an increase in unbound warfarin concentrations.

The major drug interaction effects that occur are bleeding and drugs that cause major interaction are Abicimab, amiodarone, cefepime, cefixime, Clopidogrel, Clarithromycin, econazole, erythromycin, azithromycin, caffeine, acetaminophen, tramadol, ascorbic acid, citric acid, sodium bicarbonate, ferrous sulfate, ferrous fumarate, amoxicillin, clavulanic acid, ampicillin, adalimumab, atorvastatin, amlodipine, aliskiren, acarbose, levofloxacin. [2][3][4]

Food Interactions

The common food interactions may occur with Garlic, Grape Fruit, Vit k, Vit E, Vit A, Vit C, iron-rich food, caffeine, Alcohol, Soya formula proteins, vegetable oils to be avoided. In case of eternal tube feedings, it is recommended to be given 1 hour before or after the administration of drug. [2][4][10]

Disease Interactions

The disease interactions may lead to Bleeding, Hypertension, Liver, Diabetes, Renal dysfunction. [2][4][8]

Acitrom in Comparison with Warfarin –

- Shorter half-life 10-16 hrs
- More rapid onset of action on PT
- Shorter duration of action (2days)
- Causes GI disturbances, oral ulceration and dermatitis

Adherence missed doses

If the INR is high or low, the patient may not be adhering to the regimen. Confirm the actual dose taken: if the INR is high you want to rule out the possibility that the patient took a higher than the prescribed dose. Also, always ask patients about missing any doses of warfarin. In general, a missed dose of warfarin is reflected in the INR within about 2 to 5 days after the dose is missed. This could be important even if the INR value is in the therapeutic range.

Future Trends

This is an exciting time in oral anticoagulation management. Patient self-management may be an option for patients who are very adherent and capable. Handheld instruments are available that measure the INR with sufficient accuracy, and studies show that patients can learn to manage their anticoagulation therapy after several hours of teaching, leading to improved anticoagulation control and fewer adverse events. Besides, the ease of use and availability of these instruments and computer programs to manage patients on warfarin not only has increased the use of point-of-care testing in existing anticoagulation clinics but also has led to the establishment of new clinics. This model, where face-to-face interaction occurs using point-of-care testing, is termed the near-patient testing model. So far there is little evidence the near-patient testing model leads to better outcomes than a telephone-based anticoagulation service. However, at our institution, where we manage patients in both these models, it is our experience that quicker, more efficient care is possible in the near-patient testing model. There may also be an opportunity for reimbursement using this model, whereas none is available for telephone management. We are currently undertaking a study to evaluate these two models. New antithrombotic agents are also being developed. Some parenteral direct thrombin inhibitors (DTIs) are already FDA-approved for heparin-induced thrombocytopenia, and oral DTIs are under investigation. One such DTI is ximelagatran (Exanta), which is currently being compared with warfarin and other anticoagulants in phase II and III clinical trials. This drug has shown initial promise, and if the trials show similar efficacy and safety for preventing thromboembolism in conditions such as atrial fibrillation and venous thromboembolism, this drug may ultimately start to replace warfarin because of its advantages, ie, no need for monitoring and fewer drug interactions. However, it will be a while until warfarin is replaced in clinical PR.

Chapter - 2
Review of Literatures

Xingang Li et **al, Assessment of patients warfarin knowledge and anticoagulation control at a joint physician and pharmacist managed clinic at china.** They aimed to identify the factors that significantly influence anticoagulant control. Patient's knowledge of warfarin was assessed using a validated anticoagulant knowledge assessment (AKA) questionnaire and analysis of the AKA responses was used to identify the areas for improvement in patient education. They found that the INR outcome measures "time in therapeutic range" is positively associated with patient's warfarin knowledge and educational levels among the patients, of the clinic and pharmacist, should spend more time to educate patients with a low level of education and warfarin knowledge. [11]

Elaine Othilia Yl Tang et al, conducted a study entitled **"Evaluate the patient's knowledge of warfarin and its relationship to anticoagulation."** They started the study from January to March 1999, 122 patients attending the warfarin clinic of the Prince of Wales Hospital in Hong Kong were interviewed. Their knowledge of warfarin therapy and adherence to medical advice were tested by 9 questions. A score (maximum 1.0) was calculated for each patient. And they found that 56 men and 66 women participated in the study. 60 patients (49.2 %) had read the information booklet on warfarin and had better knowledge than those who had not. Hence they concluded their study by stating that Patients' warfarin knowledge, a determinant of anticoagulation control, was generally poor. More attention should be given to the education of elderly and illiterate patients. [12]

YE MANG et al, conducted **a** study entitled **"Knowledge, satisfaction, and concerns regarding warfarin therapy and their association with warfarin adherence and anticoagulation control".** To understand patients' knowledge, satisfaction and concerns and find shortfall and help develop targeted patient education. And they established that 183 patients participated in the survey. Patients had inadequate knowledge of warfarin-diet and warfarin-drug interactions. Over 40% of the patients were not satisfied with the waiting time to see a pharmacist. The most common concerns of taking warfarin were worries about warfarin-drug interactions (36.1%), forgetting to take warfarin (26.2%) and worries about side effects (25.7%). Having Better knowledge, higher satisfaction, fewer concerns, and better warfarin adherence were associated with good INR control. [13]

Sweta Shrestha et al, have performed a present cross-sectional study entitled as **"Evaluation of patients' knowledge on warfarin in an outpatient pharmacy of a tertiary care cardiac centre".** Out of interviewing 34 patients on warfarin with a validated Anticoagulation Knowledge Assessment (AKA) questionnaire comprising 29 questions. Each correct answer scored 3.45 points whereas an incorrect answer scored 0 points. A patient who answered at least 21 questions correctly was considered to have an adequate level of knowledge or have obtained a passing score.ON tabulating the list they found that out of the 34 patients, only 5.8 % achieved a passing score whereas 94.1 % failed to achieve the passing score. 67.6 % of the patients achieved a score below 50 %. More than 50 % of the patients incorrectly answered 15 questions in the questionnaire. None of the patients scored 100 %. Warfarin knowledge was poor among the patients. Hence, regular counselling with a timely assessment of their understanding was felt necessary. [14]

Elise Schapkaitz et al, did a study entitled " **Conservative Management of Overanticoagulation in Patients With Low-Moderate Risk for Bleeding Complications**" this was a study of an average of 1500 patients attending academic hospital at the Charlotte Maxeke Johannesburg Academic Hospital (CMJAH). Patients consist of the following indications: 25% with mechanical valve replacements (MVRs) on lifelong anticoagulation therapy, 20% with a history of venous thromboembolism (VTE), and 35% anticoagulated for prevention of arterial embolism due to atrial fibrillation (AF) and 195 patients with episodes, 161 patients received conservative management. Hence they concluded that this study supports the conservative management of outpatients with INR 5 and a low–moderate risk for bleeding complications with interruption of warfarin therapy and reinstitution once the INR has decreased to the therapeutic range. [15]

Jennifer W. Baker et al, did a study entitled **INR Goal Attainment and Oral Anticoagulation Knowledge of Patients Enrolled in an Anticoagulation Clinic in a Veterans Affairs Medical Center.** They assessed the Anticoagulation knowledge 2 steps: total AKA score and count of correct answers to 15 AKA questions relevant to INR control. And they found that out of 260 participants 185 patients completed were successful. The majority of patients were undergoing anticoagulation treatment for atrial fibrillation or deep venous/pulmonary thromboembolism. The majority of patients had been treated with warfarin for at least 1 year. Most patients had goal INR ranges of 2.0 to 3.0. Of the 185 patients who completed the questionnaire, 137 achieved a passing score. The mean AKA questionnaire score was 78.1%. [16]

Sireen Abdul Rahim Shilbayeh et al, did a study entitled, **"Validation of knowledge and adherence assessment tools among patients on warfarin therapy in a Saudi hospital anticoagulant clinic".** the author did a cross-sectional survey were Patients' knowledge about warfarin was rated using an Arabic-language tool (AKA questionnaire). 52 patients were classified as having unsatisfactory knowledge. This study revealed a high prevalence of nonadherence and poor knowledge in the population[17]

Ebru baysal et al, Effects of structured patient education on the knowledge level and INR control of patients receiving warfarin: Randomized Controlled Trial To determine the effects of patient education about the safety of warfarin therapy on related knowledge levels and International Normalized Ratio (INR) control. Participants in the intervention group received one-to-one education about the safety of warfarin therapy and a booklet. Participants in the control group received usual care. Patients' warfarin knowledge levels in both groups were measured three times at monthly intervals. Before education, warfarin knowledge levels were inadequate in the intervention group, but it was higher after education and reached a good level.No significant difference was found between the International Normalized Ratio controls of the two groups. No significant relationship was found between pre- and post-education warfarin knowledge levels and the INR number in the therapeutic range. One-to-one education supported by written and visual material was effective in increasing patients' warfarin knowledge levels. [18]

Leili Pourafkari et al, conducted a study entitled"**Factors Influencing Various Aspects of Patients' Knowledge of Oral Anticoagulation**" the author enrolled patients treated using warfarin for anticoagulation during 6 months at a university-affiliated cardiac clinic. All demographic and clinical information were collected and (AKA) questionnaire consisting of 29 questions was used to interview. Out of 150 (79 men and 71 women) with a median age of 61.5 years completed the AKA questionnaire. The average overall score was 29.3%. The author concluded that the Socioeconomic factors and level of general education are the most important elements determining the patient awareness of therapeutic goals[19]

Salihah Aidit et al, conducted a study entitled **"Effect of Standardized Warfarin Treatment Protocol on Anticoagulant Effect: Comparison of a Warfarin Medication Therapy Adherence Clinic with Usual Medical Care"** the author intended a retrospective cohort study was in a cardiology referral hospital located in central Kuala Lumpur, Malaysia, from 2009 to 2014. Out of 473 patients, 151 patients fulfilled the inclusion criteria. The findings revealed that there were significant associations between the usual medical care (UMC) group and pharmacist-led WMTAC in terms of TTR and INR levels. A positive impact of pharmacists' involvement in the WMTAC clinic was where the "pharmacist's recommendation accepted and expanded therapeutic INR range" were statistically significantly higher in the WMTAC group. There was a significant positive association between the pharmacist-led WMTAC and anticoagulation effect (therapeutic TTR, INR). The identified findings revealed that the expanded role of the pharmacist in pharmacist-managed warfarin therapy is beneficial to optimize warfarin therapy. This study also highlighted the critical roles that pharmacists can actively play to ensure optimal anticoagulation pharmaceutical[20]

Ravindra Nath Sahay et al, conducted a study entitled *"Study of environmental and genetic factors determining warfarin toxicity".* The author stated that the study is to determine age, gender, pharmacogenetics, drugs influencing warfarin toxicity in Indian patients. The most common age for Warfarin toxicity in our study was between 30 to 39 years (22.5%) with a mean of 42.9 years. Bleeding risk was higher in the elderly with 14 out of 26 patients with age >50 years had bleeding manifestations. Toxicity was more prevalent in female (60%). 40% patients were on drugs interacting with warfarin; NSAIDS (Nonsteroidal Anti-Inflammatory Drug) and antibiotics were the most common interacting drugs. In our study, 17.5% of patients had acute liver disease and one patient had deranged creatinine (2.6). 40% of patients had VKORC1 variants and 35% of patients had CYP2C9 variants. Maximum patients developed toxicity within 15-30 days of initiation of warfarin. The author concluded that warfarin toxicity has a multifactorial cause. Drugs and Genetic variation are the most common factors influencing warfarin toxicity. Warfarin toxicity has a low mortality rate, although it increases with (International Normalised Ratio) INR>10 and with increasing age. [21]

Doris Barcellona et al, conducted a study entitled *"Patient education and oral anticoagulant therapy"*. *The author explained about* The stability of oral anticoagulant therapy is affected by an irregular intake of vegetables, interactions with other drugs, intercurrent disease, and compliance. Intending to investigate whether educating patients could affect anticoagulation stability, we prepared a questionnaire based on some fundamental information given by us to our patients during their first attendance to our clinic. The questionnaire was administered to a group of 219 anticoagulated patients attending our Thrombosis Center. All patients were invited to fill in the questionnaire, which was handed out by a nurse, while they were waiting for their blood sampling results. None of the patients refused to fill in the questionnaire, which was completed at once and independently. The answers to the questionnaire were correlated with the time spent by the patients in the therapeutic range. A significant difference was found between the time spent in the therapeutic range by patients who declared a regular intake of their therapy (91%, 14-100%) and that spent in the range by those who answered they sometimes forgot to take it (75%, 9-100%). The percentage of time spent in the therapeutic range was significantly longer (92%, 36%-100%) in patients who reported regular vegetable intake and in those that never ate vegetables than that observed in patients who admitted occasional intake of vegetables (86%, 5%-100%). The author concluded that: 1) that greater emphasis should be given to educational courses for anticoagulated patients especially in consideration of age and gender differences, and 2) on its own, administration of the questionnaire leads to a significant improvement in the time spent by patients in the therapeutic range. [22]

Jean-François Chenot et al, conducted a study entitled *"Safety relevant knowledge of orally anticoagulated patients without self-monitoring".* The author stated about the aim of this study was to assess patient knowledge about OAT and factors associated with patient knowledge. This is a baseline survey of a cluster-randomized controlled trial in 22 general practices with an educational intervention for patients or their caregivers. We assessed knowledge about general information on OAT and key facts regarding nutrition, drug interactions and other safety precautions of 345 patients at baseline. The results explained that Half of the participants (49%) were unaware of dietary recommendations. The majority (80%) did not know which non-prescription analgesic is the safest and 73% indicated they would not inform pharmacists about OAT. Many participants (35-75%) would not recognize important emergencies. After adjustment in a multivariate analysis, older age and less than 10 years education remained significantly associated with a lower overall score, but not with self-rated knowledge. The author concluded that the patients have relevant knowledge gaps, potentially affecting safe and effective OAT. There is a need to assess patient knowledge and for structured education programs. (23)

Miho Kimachi et al, conducted a study entitled *"Direct oral anticoagulants versus warfarin for preventing stroke and systemic embolic events among atrial fibrillation patients with chronic kidney disease".* The author conducted a study to assess the efficacy and safety of DOAC including apixaban, dabigatran, edoxaban, and rivaroxaban versus warfarin among AF patients with CKD. Two review authors independently selected studies, assessed quality, and extracted data. They calculated the risk ratio (RR) and 95% confidence intervals (95% CI) for the association between anticoagulant therapy and all strokes and systemic embolic events as the primary efficacy outcome and major bleeding events as the primary safety outcome. Confidence in the evidence was assessed using GRADE. Study duration ranged from 1.8 to 2.8 years. The large majority of participants included in this study were CKD stage G3 (12,155), and a small number were stage G4 (390). Of 12,545 participants from five studies, a total of 321 cases (2.56%) of the primary efficacy outcome occurred per year. Further, of 12,521 participants from five studies, a total of 617 cases (4.93%) of the primary safety outcome occurred per year. DOAC appeared to probably reduce the incidence of stroke and systemic embolism events (5 studies, 12,545 participants: RR 0.81, 95% CI 0.65 to 1.00; moderate certainty evidence) and to slightly reduce the incidence of major bleeding events (5 studies, 12,521 participants: RR 0.79, 95% CI 0.59 to 1.04; low certainty evidence) in comparison with warfarin. The author concluded that the findings indicated that DOAC is as likely as warfarin to prevent all strokes and systemic embolic events without increasing risk of major bleeding events among AF patients with kidney impairment. [24]

Anne Sig Vestergaard et al, conducted a study entitled *"The importance of mean time in therapeutic range for complication rates in warfarin therapy of patients with atrial fibrillation".* The author explained the correlation between TTR and the occurrence of complications during warfarin therapy has been established, but the influence of patient characteristics in that respect remains undetermined. The objective of the present papers was to examine the association between mean TTR and complication rates with adjustment for differences in relevant patient cohort characteristics. The association between the reported mean TTR and major bleeding and stroke/systemic embolism was analyzed by random-effects meta-regression with and without adjustment for relevant clinical cohort characteristics. In the adjusted meta-regressions, the impact of mean TTR on the occurrence of hemorrhage was adjusted for the mean age and the proportion of populations with prior stroke or transient ischemic attack. In the adjusted analyses on thromboembolism, the proportion of females was, furthermore, included. The results estimated that out of 2169 papers, 35 papers met pre-specified inclusion criteria, holding relevant information on 31 patient cohorts. In univariable meta-regression, increasing mean TTR was significantly associated with a decreased rate of both major bleeding and stroke/systemic embolism. However, after adjustment mean TTR was no longer significantly associated with stroke/systemic embolism. The author concluded that mainly the safety of warfarin therapy increases with higher mean TTR, whereas effectiveness appears not to be substantially improved. [25]

Deeplakshmi M et al, conducted a study entitled *"A New Point-Of-Care Monitoring Service by Community Pharmacists in India".* The author implemented an INR monitoring service by community pharmacists for optimizing the therapy outcomes of Warfarin, used widely for its anticoagulant activity both as a treatment and prophylaxis. The study was conducted in selected community pharmacies associated with general practitioners. The patients in the intervention arm received point of care INR measurement and anticoagulant management including assessment of clinical and quality of life endpoints by their pharmacists in collaboration with their general practitioners. From the study, it was revealed that about 44 % (n = 36) of the patients recruited into the intervention group submitted their retrospective INR reports which were considered as pre-intervention data and used to compare the clinical outcome against post-intervention phases. It was found that the patients in the post-intervention group had a statistically significant ($p < 0.05$) control in the INR values than the pre-intervention group. A statistically significant difference ($p = 0.025$) was observed in the quality of life of patients at pre and post-intervention groups. There was also a significant ($p = 0.016$) increase in patient's knowledge about anticoagulant therapy between pre and post-intervention. The author concluded that the community pharmacists and medical practitioners managed anticoagulant service is feasible and acceptable to patients and pharmacist involved in the study. [26]

Laila Mahmoud Matalqah et al, conducted a study entitled *"a translation and validation study of the Oral Anticoagulation Knowledge (OAK) Test".* The author stated that there is no validated knowledge assessment tool to examine the relationship between patient knowledge regarding warfarin therapy and it's safe and effective in Malaysia. The main objective is to translate the Oral Anticoagulation Knowledge (OAK) Test into the Malay language (Bahasa Malaysia) and to examine the psychometric properties of the Malaysian version. In a prospective, parallel-group study, 382 consecutive outpatients with atrial fibrillation prescribed warfarin treatment were identified. And also there were certain criteria, according to it, patients were selected for the study. Patients who had severe health problems or cognitive impairment and could not complete interviews were excluded. A standard translation procedure was used to develop the Malaysian version of the

OAK from the original English version. Face-to-face interviews included administration of the translated 20-question test and a collection of socio-demographic data. Medical records were reviewed for INR levels and other clinical data. Only 215 were eligible and accepted to complete the questionnaires. The mean±SD of OAK scores was 47.6±17.6. Good internal consistency was found (Cronbach's alpha = 0.767); the test-retest reliability value was 0.871 (p<0.001). For known group validity, a significant relationship between OAK categories and TTR (INR) categories (chi-square = 12.24; p <0.05) was found. The author concluded that OAK is a reliable and valid measure of Warfarin knowledge that may be a useful tool for research and clinical practice. There is a need for improvement in patient education, including reinforcement of dietary guidelines for warfarin therapy. [27]

Sahimi Mohamed et al, conducted a study entitled *"Development of Knowledge of Anticoagulant Questionnaire".* The author stated that this study aimed to develop a new instrument to measure KAC among the Malaysian population. The items for the new KAC-Q were developed based on the narrative literature review and focus group discussion. The Delphi Method was used to assess the content validity of the new KAC-Q. Fifteen experts were involved in three phases of the Delphi survey. The face validity was examined to ensure that the items in the questionnaire were understood by the targeted patients. The results revealed that the items for new KAC-Q were developed based on the narrative literature review and focus group discussion. The Delphi Method was used to assess the content validity of the new KAC-Q. Fifteen experts were involved in three phases of the Delphi survey. The face validity was examined to ensure that the items in the questionnaire were understood by the targeted patients. The author concluded that with good structured and adequate information, these 28 KAC-Q questions were considered to have good content and face validity. However, further psychometric testing is needed to ensure that KAC-Q is reliable and valid to aid health care providers in determining patients' anticoagulant knowledge in targeted populations. [28]

Sandip Jadav et al, conducted a study entitled **"Utilization Pattern of Antiplatelet and Anticoagulant Medicines Among the Patients Suffering From Atrial Fibrillation".** The author explained the Primary objective was to study the usage pattern of antiplatelet and anticoagulant drugs in AF patients. The secondary objective was to assess the risk of stroke and compare usage pattern of antithrombotic drugs in non-valvular atrial fibrillation (NVAF) patients with application of CHADS2 and CHA2DS2-VASc score. A prospective and observational study was conducted in outpatient department for one year in patients > 35 years of either gender diagnosed with AF due to any established cause. CHADS2 and CHA2DS2-VASc score were used to assess the risk of stroke among NVAF patients. The results showed that 111 patients diagnosed with AF (mean age 54 years; 54.96% female) were analyzed and out of these, 78 patients were valvular AF patients and 33 were NVAF patients. Anticoagulants were predominantly prescribed in 60 valvular AF patients. Out of 33 NVAF patients, 19

(57.57%) patients had CHADS2 score 1 while as per CHA2DS2-VASc score 28 (84.84%) patients had score ≥ 2. Out of 33 NVAF patients, 15 (45.45%) patients were prescribed warfarin, aspirin in 12 (36.36%) patients and no antithrombotic therapy in 6 (18.18%) patients. The author concluded that oral anticoagulant drugs are most commonly prescribed antithrombotic drugs in valvular AF and NVAF patients for stroke prevention. CHADS2 and CHA2DS2-VASc score are easy, simple schemes to assess stroke risk in NVAF patients and helps physicians and patients to choose the most suitable antithrombotic therapy. [29]

A.L. Briggs et al, conducted a study entitled *"The development and performance validation of a tool to assess patient anticoagulation knowledge".* The author explained the patient-specific medication management education and functions as a tool for continuous quality improvement in anticoagulation education. Using objective measurement methods, a convenience sample of 60 English-speaking patients receiving services from an inner-city and suburban pharmacist managed anticoagulation clinics were used in conjunction with objective measurement methods. Rasch analysis of 32 multiple-choice items representing 10 anticoagulation educational content areas demonstrated misfit statistics of less than 1.2. All 60 patients demonstrated person misfit statistics of less than 1.3. The educational content area was well represented and distributed. The author concluded that because the AKA performed well, the data support that information gained from the AKA will provide pharmacists with direction for anticoagulation management education that is targeted to each patient's specific needs. Additionally, responses demonstrated objective data about those components of practice that are being taught effectively. [30]

Chapter- 3

Need for the study

Warfarin is a widely used anticoagulant with a narrow therapeutic index, and it requires close monitoring and adequate patient education. We aimed to assess the knowledge level regarding warfarin therapy among its users and to identify the factors that significantly influence anticoagulation control.

Our objective was also to investigate the relationships between anticoagulant knowledge, health literacy, and self-reported adherence in patients taking warfarin and directly acting oral anticoagulants.

Need for the Stduy

Patient's Knowledge Assessment on Vitamin K Antagonist

Chapter- 4

Plan of Work

Tools

a) Socio-Demographic Details –

- These details include all the socio-demographic details, such as –

  age, gender, height, weight, etc.

- Medical history, clinical and treatment-related details are collected from patient case profile.

- PT INR report

- (anticoagulation knowledge assessment) AKA questionnaire.

- The Prescription data was analyzed based on details - several drugs, names of individual drugs, dose, dosage form, dosing schedule (acitrom, warfarin).

b) Study Procedure -

- The data will be collected at the regular outpatient department.

- Standard data entry format was used and prescriptions were individually screened to assess the drug interactions.

- Data source needed for the study was collected from care reports, treatment charts and lab reports.

c) Materials

Data Collection Forms: Anticoagulation knowledge assessment questionnaire is designed for recording the parameters.

The content of the verbal education includes the following –

- Warfarin/Acitrom therapy (treatment rationale, benefits, and length).
- Medication administration (dosing, when to take a dose, how to store the medication, and what to do in case of a missed dose).
- Drug-drug or drug-food interactions.
- Dietary considerations and consistency.
- Side effects (signs of over-anticoagulation or disease recurrence, and what to do in case of bleeding).
- Laboratory monitoring (INR and frequency).

Statistical Analysis:

All the experimental values were expressed as Mean standard deviation and percentage.

Chapter- 5

Aims and Objectives

Aim

The aims of this study are –

- To assess the knowledge level of patients receiving warfarin / acitrom therapy in a hospital by using the validated Anticoagulation Knowledge Assessment (AKA) questionnaire.
- To examine the relationship between patients' warfarin / acitrom knowledge and anticoagulant control as measured by the INR.

Objective

- To assess the patient knowledge and barriers to warfarin / acitrom medication usage
- To prevent non-adherence and wrong practices of patients

Patient's Knowledge Assessment on Vitamin K Antagonist

Chapter- 6
Methodology

---

a) Study Site:

The study is conducted at the CARE hospital, Banjara Hills, Hyderabad, a tertiary care hospital.

b) Study Design:

This is a prospective, Knowledge, Attitude, and Practice (KAP) study.

c) Study Duration:

Six months.

d) Selection of Patient:

Inclusion Criteria:

All age groups are included, both male and female genders with class 1 indication of Vit K Antagonist

Exclusive Criteria:

1) Subjects who are not willing to participate

2) Subjects with incomplete data

3) Subjects without the indication of vitamin k antagonist

The present study involves the process of assessing the knowledge of patients about ways of using vitamin k antagonist with a validated AKA which was prescribed in care hospital, Banjara hills.

The study involves the following steps.

1. Collection of prescriptions.
2. Interviewing the patients with the AKA Questionnaire
3. Analysing the prescription and it's lab investigations to know the INR Control.

Collection of Prescriptions:

A total of 100 cases were collected in the electrophysiology department, care hospital, Banjara hills for 6 months.

Interviewing the Patients with the AKA Questionnaire:

Patient details of each case sheet-like prescription and lab investigations were noted in the AKA. Proforma includes age, name, sex, diagnosis, chief complaints, drugs, Drug-drug interactions, lab investigations, practices followed by patients while using the drug-like regular patient's check-up, following of diet restriction.

Analysing the Prescription and it's Lab Investigations to know the INR Control:

The patient prescriptions and lab data were analysed for their adherence to the therapy and INR control.

Chapter- 7

Results and Discussion

This is knowledge, attitude and practice prospective study in which we evaluate the relationship between knowledge of patients about vitamin k antagonist and their INR control

A total number of cases (N=100) were screened during the study period

The data of the patients were categorised according to age, gender, other causes of lack of INR control, causality assessment. The percentages were calculated according to the figures described.

From the total of 100 cases, all the patient's knowledge has been screened, in which INR control cases were found to be n= 27, whereas the interventional cases were found to be n=73 which is summarized in table no:7.1 and figure no:7.1

Table 7.1: Study Population

S. No	Study Population	Number of Cases	Percentage
1	Control group	27	27%
2	Interventional group	73	73%
3	Total number of cases	100	100%

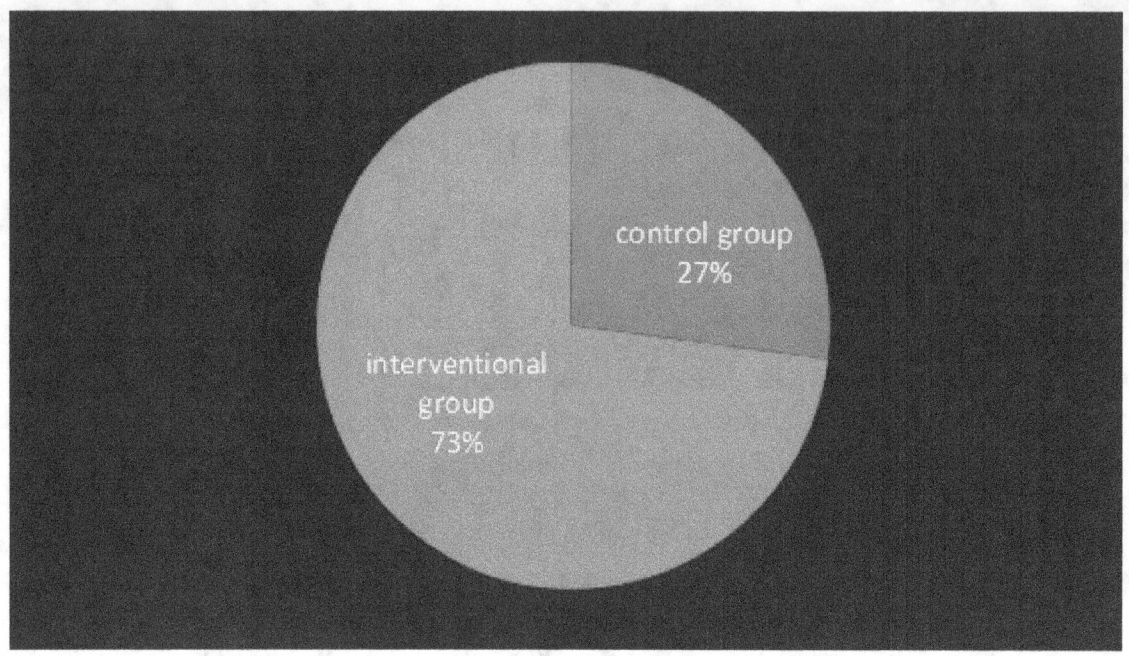

Fig 7.1: Graphical Representation of Study Population

Summary of baseline characteristics of study patients

The basic characters of patients in the study group are given in Table 7.2

Table 7.2: Basic Characters of Patients in the Study Group

Characteristics	Interventional group	Control group
Male patients	36	15
Female patients	37	12
Patients with no comorbidity	10	5
Age 30-40	13	5
Age 41-50	20	10
Age 51-60	30	10
Above 60	10	2
Ethnicity	Asian	Asian

Patient's Knowledge Assessment on Vitamin K Antagonist

Gender Distribution in Interventional Group

Among 73 cases of an interventional group, the total number of male patients were found to be 49.32% (n=36) and female patients were found to be 50.32% (n=37) given in table7.3, figure7.2

Table 7.3: Gender Distribution in Interventional Group

Gender	Percentage	Number
Male	49.32%	36
Female	50.68%	37
Total patients	100%	73

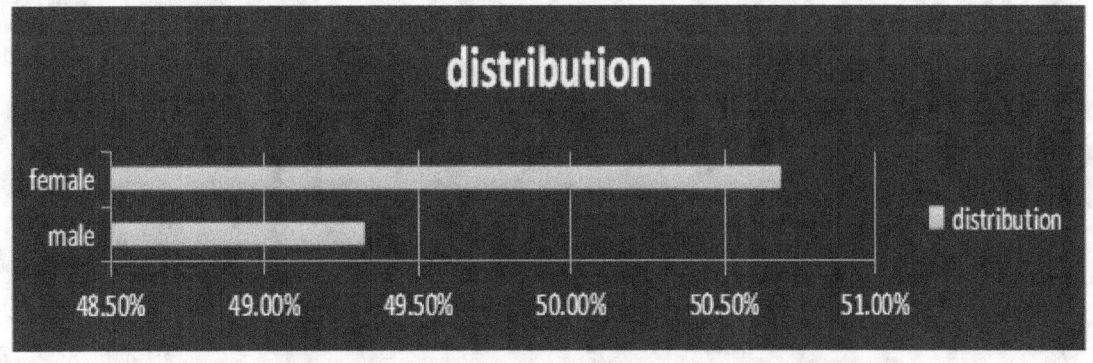

Fig7.2: Gender Distribution in Interventional Group

Causes of Intervention in INR Control

In this study, it has been found that 4 major causes that lead to intervention in INR control which includes drug-drug interactions, food-drug interactions, economic background, lack of knowledge which is mentioned in table 7.4 and figure 7.3

Table 7.4: Causes of Intervention in INR Control

Cause	Number	Percentage
Drug-Drug Interactions	5	7%
Food-Drug Interactions	6	8%
Lack of Knowledge	57	78%
Economic Background	5	7%
Total Interventional Group	73	100%

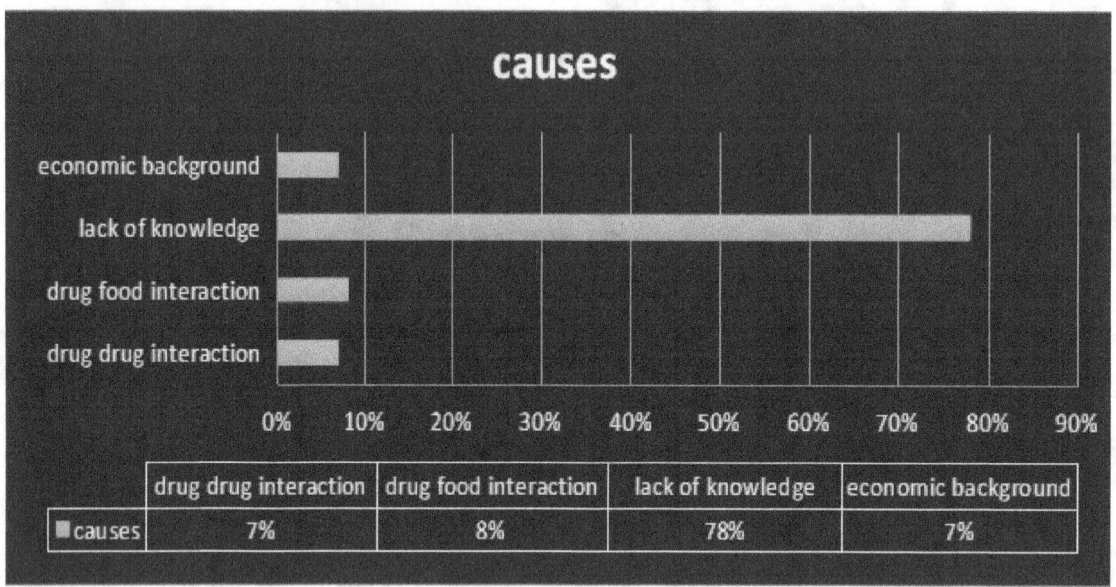

Fig 7.3: Causes of intervention in INR control

Drug-drug interaction

From a total of 73 cases, drug-drug interactions were found to be in 5 patients. These 5 patients interacted individually with a specific area of drugs such as herbal medications and OTC medications. The numbers of drug interacting cases were mentioned in table number 7.4. Two main kinds of a drug interaction that can be included were OTC medication interaction and herbal medication interaction, which is mentioned in table 7.5 and fig 7.4and fig7.5

Table 7.5: Two Main Kind of Drug Interaction

Drugs interacting	Percentage	No. of patients
Herbal medication	60%	3
OTC medication	40%	2
Total population	100%	5

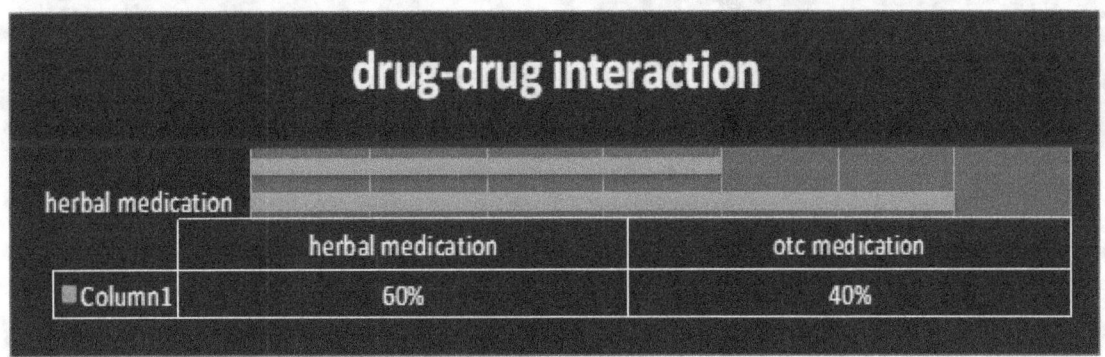

Fig 7.4: Two Main kind of Drug Interaction

Food-Drug Interaction

From a total of 73 cases, food-drug interactions were found to be in 6 patients. These 6 patients interacted individually with specific food types such as greens, leafy vegetables and proteins. The numbers of food interacting cases were mentioned in table number 7.4. Main kinds of food interaction are vitamin k rich food like greens, leafy vegetables and proteins. Given in Table 1.6 and fig 1.5

Table 7.6: Kinds of Food Interaction

Food interaction	Percentage	No. of patients
Greens and leafy Vegetables	83%	5
Proteins	17%	1
Total no patients	100%	6

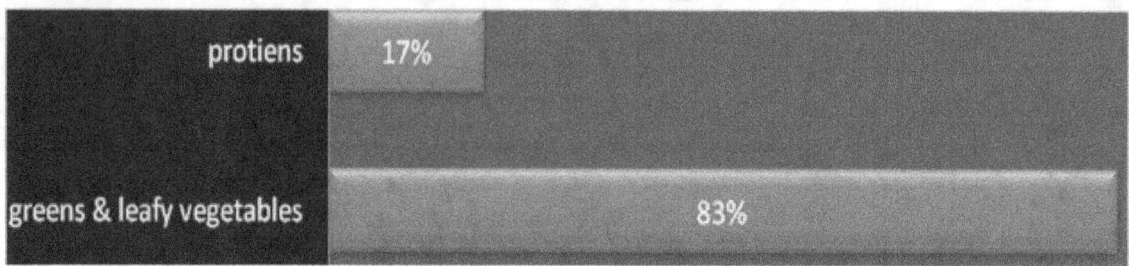

Fig 7.5: Kinds of Food Interaction

Patients Knowledge Scoring

- Patients passed with 100% knowledge are 4% (n=4)

- Patients passed with passing score or above are 23%(n=23)

- Patients failed are 73% (n=73)

- INR control was found to be 27% (n=27%) as Given in fig 7.6

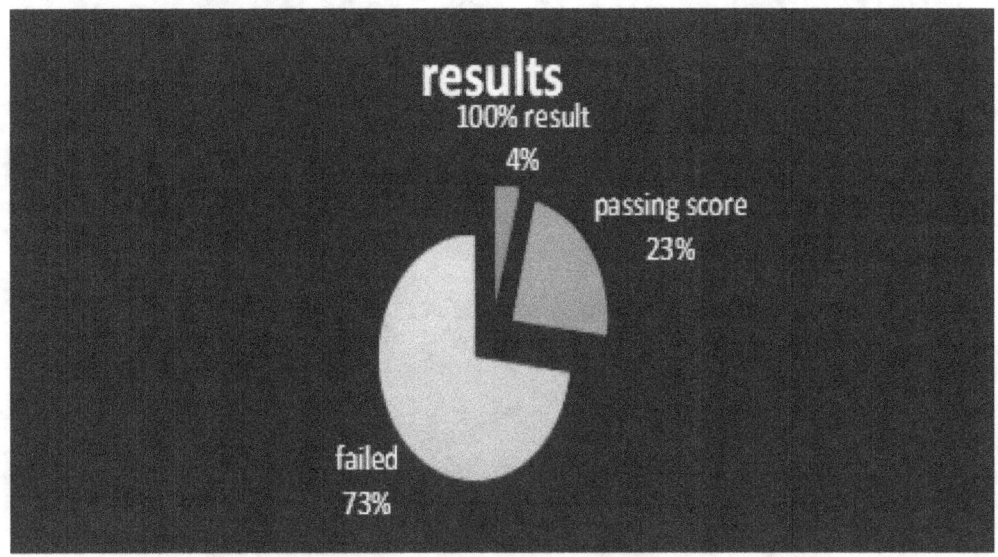

Fig 7.6: Patients Knowledge Scoring

INR Deviations of Interventional Patients

Among the 73 interventional patients the INR deviation can be either lower (<1.7) to target INR or higher (>3.5) to target INR. The INR deviation percentage is given in the below table 1.7 and figure1.7

Table 7.7: INR Deviation

INR deviations	Interventional patients	Percentage
Lower to Target	52	71.3%
Higher to Target	21	28.7%
Total no. of Interventional Patients	73	100%

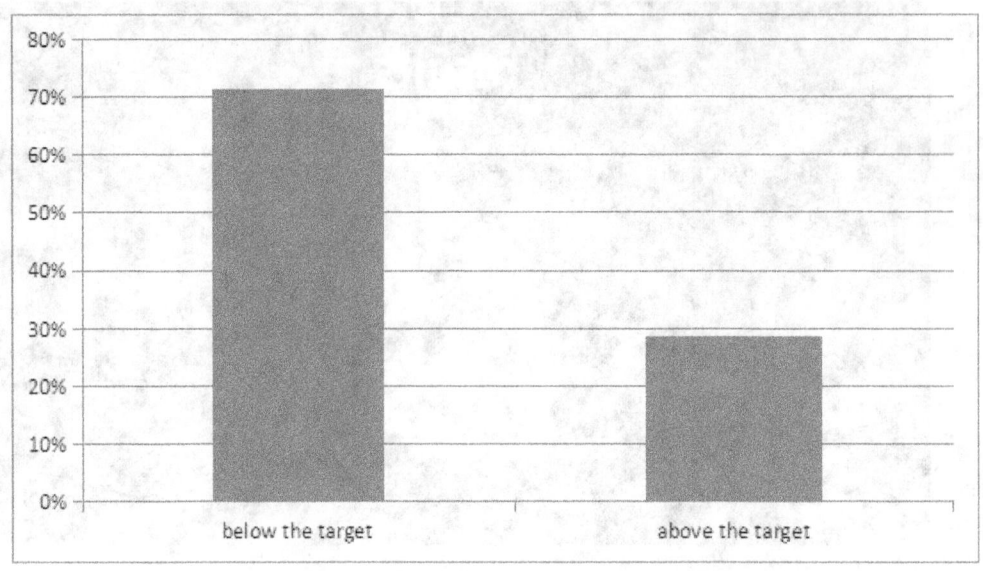

Fig 7.7: INR Deviation

ADRs Faced by Interventional Patients

4 main ADRs can be faced in anticoagulation studies such as bleeding in gums, bloody stools, gastrointestinal discomfort, and rash. As given in table 1.8, figure 1.8

Table 7.8: ADRs Faced by Interventional Patients

ADRs	Percentage	No of patients
Gastrointestinal Discomfort	28%	7
Rash	12%	3
Blood in Gums	36%	9
Bloody Stools	24%	6
Interventional Patients Faced ADRs	100%	25

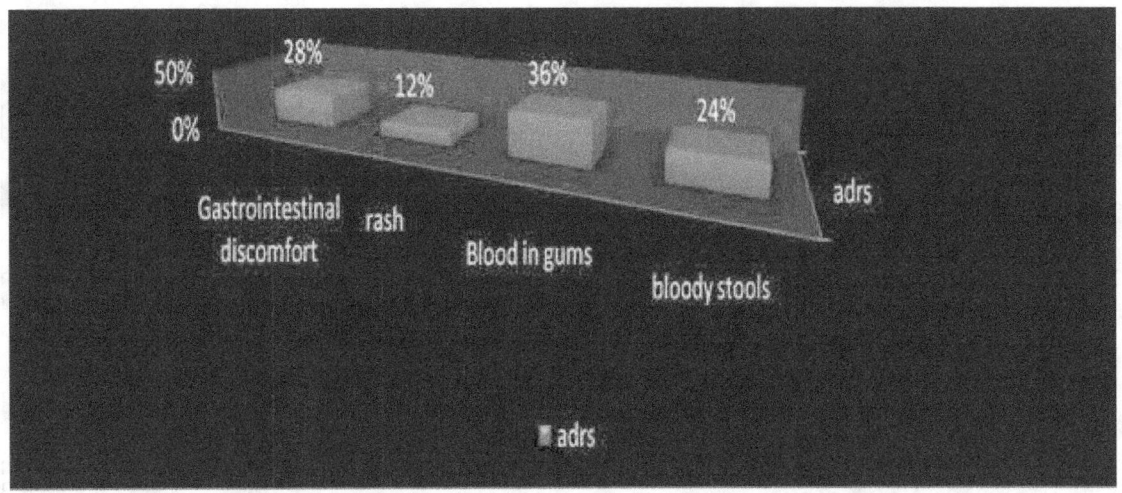

Fig 7.8: ADRs Faced by Interventional Patients

Patients Scoring Based on Each Question

Table 7.9: Patients Knowledge Based on Scoring

S. No	Question	No. of patients	percentage
1	Coumadin (warfarin) may be used to	100	100%
2	Any of the healthcare providers must tell him/her in case he/she does not know about your treatment	33	33%
3	The PT/INR test is	100	100%
4	A patient with knowledge of PT/INR safe range	100	100%
5	The best thing to do if you miss a dose of warfarin is to?	25	25%
6	A patient with knowledge about an emergency	100	100%
7	When is it safe to take a medication that interacts with warfarin?	23	23%
8	Taking a medication containing aspirin while on warfarin will	10	10%

9	A patient on warfarin therapy should contact the physician or healthcare provider who monitors it when?	90	90%
10	Which of the following vitamins interacts with warfarin	72	72%
11	Which of the following vitamins interacts with warfarin	63	63%
12	Occasionally eating a large amount of leafy greens vegetables while taking warfarin can?	23	23%

Discussion

The study was carried out in 100 patients, out of which 27% (n=27) have good INR control and 73% (n=73) patients have interventional INR. Among this interventional population, 73% (n=52) have low INR and 28.7% (n=21) have higher INR based on the target INR.

This population has 49.32% (n=36) are male and 50.68 (n=37) are female

The study population that faced 4 main ADRs such as bleeding in gums, bloody stools, gastrointestinal discomfort, the rash was 34.2% (n=25)

Based on the knowledge the scoring of the population was

• Patients passed with 100% knowledge are 4% (n=4)

• Patients passed with passing score or above are 23% (n=23)

- Patients failed are 73% (n=73)

- INR control was found to be 27% (n=27%)

The lack of INR control due to drug-drug interaction was found to be 5% (n=5) and the lack of INR control due to drug-food interaction was found to be 6% (n=6)

The other reasons that remained are lack of knowledge 57% (n=57) and economic background and affordability 5% (n=5)

There is no age and comorbidity bias in this study as age doesn't contribute to INR control as well the comorbidity

The results help us make a statement that INR control is directly proportional to the knowledge of patients. To avoid Vitamin k antagonist interventions it's important to educate the patients.

Patient's Knowledge Assessment on Vitamin K Antagonist

Chapter-8
Summary

Vitamin K Antagonist (VKA)

VKA is a blood thinner prescribed to prevent and treat blood clots. This therapy may be prescribed for patients with certain types of irregular heartbeat, blood clots in the legs or lungs, and patients who have certain medical device implants such as artificial heart valves. They are a group of substances that reduce blood clotting by reducing the action of vitamin K dependent clotting factor. They are used as anticoagulant medications in the prevention of thrombosis. Examples – Coumadin (Warfarin), (jantoven), Acenocoumarol (nicumalon), (acitrom).

Warfarin is a widely used anticoagulant with a narrow therapeutic index, and it requires close monitoring and adequate patient education. We aimed to assess the knowledge level regarding warfarin therapy among its users and to identify the factors that significantly influence anticoagulation control.

INR test meters may be prescribed to patients for use in the home, and they may also be used by health care providers. However, India is not so famous with this practice and is also not economical for the Indian population. How often an INR is monitored and the results a patient should expect, will be based on the advice from the physician. An INR target range is typically between 2.0 and 3.0 for basic blood-thinning, anyhow the range may vary based on a patient's conditions .medication dose is changed according to INR Patients should work with their physician for achieving and maintaining a target INR.

The data will be collected using a validated Anticoagulation knowledge assessment questionnaire is designed for recording the parameters like Warfarin/Acitrom therapy (treatment rationale, benefits, and length).Medication administration (dosing, when to take a dose, how to store the medication, and what to do in case of a missed dose). Drug-drug or drug-food interactions Dietary considerations and consistency. Side effects (signs of over-anticoagulation or disease recurrence, and what to do in case of bleeding). Laboratory monitoring (INR and frequency), at the regular outpatient department of a tertiary hospital, Standard data entry format was used and prescriptions were individually screened to assess the drug interactions. Data source needed for the study was collected from care reports, treatment charts and lab reports.

Patients' knowledge of warfarin was assessed using a validated Anticoagulation Knowledge Assessment (AKA) questionnaire. Patients' responses to each question were analyzed to identify areas of improvement in current warfarin education. International normalized ratio (INR) control was defined by the time in therapeutic range (TTR).

The study has carried out 100 patients, out of which 27% (n=27) have good INR control and 73% (n=73) patients have interventional INR. Among this interventional population 72.3% (n=52) have low INR and 28.7% (n=21) have higher INR based on the target INR. This population has 49.32% (n=36) are male and 50.68 (n=37) are female. The study population that faced 4 main ADRs such as bleeding in gums, bloody stools, gastrointestinal discomfort, the rash was 34.2% (n=25).

Based on the knowledge the scoring of the population was

- Patients passed with 100% knowledge are 4% (n=4)

- Patients passed with passing score or above are 23%(n=23)

- Patients failed are 73% (n=73)

- INR control was found to be 27% (n=27%)

The lack of INR control due to drug-drug interaction was found to be 5% (n=5) and the lack of INR control due to drug-food interaction was found to be 6% (n=6). The other reasons that remained are lack of knowledge 57% (n=57) and economic background and affordability 5% (n=5). There is no age and comorbidity bias in this study as age doesn't contribute to INR control as well as the comorbidity.

The results help us make a statement that INR control is directly proportional to the knowledge of patients. To avoid VKA interventions it's important to educate the patients.

Areas for improvement in patient education have been identified, and processes for educational modification are currently in development. This survey shows that there is still room for improvement of patient education and compliance in patients treated with anticoagulants. Education of VKA patients thus should be reinforced to reduce complications rates and improve compliance. This holds in particular for patients taking OACs. There is a need for improvement in patient education, including reinforcement of dietary guidelines for warfarin therapy as well as when it is appropriate to contact the clinic for questions.

Chapter - 9
Study Limitations

Altogether 150 patients were asked to participate in the study, out of which only 100 patients (66.66 %) agreed for participation. The sample size was small to generalize the study. Large scale and multi-centric study would be mandatory to generalize the study findings, for which this study could become a pathfinder in a resource constraint country like India.

We did not collect information on the quality of education given to participants on their OACs upon initiation, nor did we determine whether participants who were taking a DOAC at the time of the interview had previously been taking warfarin. The limitations of the tools used should also be considered.

Medication adherence was quantified by self-report; this approach can overestimate the level of adherence observed.

Patient's Knowledge Assessment on Vitamin K Antagonist

References

1. Essentials of Medical Pharmacology (7th edition) by K D Tripathi.

2. Holbrook AM, Crowther NR, Hirsh J, Interactions of warfarin with drugs and food by Wells PS1, Ann Intern Med. 1994. 9th edition: 676-683.

3. www.micromedex.com/interactionchecker/warfarin/

4. www.drugs.com/drugs/warfarin

5. www.micromedex.com/drugs/warfarin

6. https://www.fda.gov/MedicalDevices/ProductsandMedicalProcedures/InVitroDiagnostics/WarfarinINRTestMeters/default.htm

7. https://crediblemeds.org/

8. http://www.heart.org/en/health-topics/arrhythmia/prevention--treatment-of-arrhythmia/a-patients-guide-to-taking-warfarin

9. https://www.nhs.uk/conditions/warfarin/

10. https://www.clinicalkey.com/#!/content/patient_handout/5-s2.0-pe_gold_standard650_226_en

11. LI   X,   SUN   S,   Wang   Q. Assessment of patients' warfarin knowledge and   anticoagulation control at a joint physician and pharmacist managed clinic in china. 2018. 12th edition: 783-791.

12. Elainethilia YL Tang, Cemen SM Lai, Kenneth KC Lee, Relationship between Patients' Warfarin Knowledge and Anticoagulation Control, Hong Kong. 2003.

13. Wang Y, Kong MC, Lee LH, Knowledge, satisfaction, and concerns regarding warfarin therapy and their association with warfarin adherence and anticoagulation control, 4th edition: 2014: 550 – 554.

14. Sweta Shrestha, Binaya Sapkot, Anjana Kumpakha, Evaluation patients' of knowledge on in warfarin outpatient pharmacy of tertiary a care cardiac centre. India. 8th edition, 2015: 429.

15. Elise Schapkaitz, Susan Louw, Jessica Friedman, et al. Conservative Management of Over anticoagulation in Patients with Low–Moderate Risk for Bleeding Complications Clinical and Applied Thrombosis/Homeostasis. 2018;24(8): 1255-1260.

16. Jennifer W Baker, Kristi L Pierce, Casey A Ryals. Goal Attainment and Oral Anticoagulation Knowledge of Patients Enrolled in Anticoagulation Clinic in a Veterans Affairs Medical Center. JMCP Journal of Managed Care Pharmacy. 2011; 17(2).

17. Sireen Abdul, Rahim Shilbayeh, Wejdan Ali Almutairi et al. Validation of knowledge and adherence assessment tools among patients on warfarin therapy in a Saudi hospital anticoagulant clinic: International Journal of Clinical Pharmacy. 2018; 40:56–66.

18. Ebru Baysal, Tulay Sagkal Midilli, et al. Effects of structured patient education on the knowledge level and INR control of patients receiving warfarin: Randomized Controlled Trial. Pak J Med Sci. 2018;34(2):240-246.

19. Leili Pourafkari, Aidin Baghbani-Oskouei, Mohammadreza Taban-Sadeghi et al. Factors Influencing Various Aspects of Patients' Knowledge of Oral Anticoagulation. Journal of Cardiovascular Pharmacology. 2018;71(3):174–179.

20. Salihah Aidit, Yee Chang Soh, Chuan Seng Yap et al. Effect of Standardized Warfarin Treatment Protocol on Anticoagulant Effect: Comparison of a Warfarin Medication Therapy Adherence Clinic with Usual Medical Care Front Pharmacol. 2017;8:637.

21. Ravindra Nath Sahay, Kaustubh Dilip Salagre, Khushali Rajesh Dedhia. Study of environmental and genetic factors determining warfarin toxicity International Journal of Research in Medical Sciences Sahay RN et al. Int J Res Med Sci. 2017;5(2):463-468.

22. Doris Barcellona, Paolo Contu, Francesco Marongiu, et al. Patient education and oral anticoagulant therap. Haematologica. 2002; 87:1081-108.

23. Jean-François Chenot, Thanh Duc Hua, Manar Abu Abed, et al. Safety relevant knowledge of orally anticoagulated patients without self-monitoring: a baseline survey in primary care. BMC Family Practice. 2014;15:104.

24. Kimachi M, Furukawa TA, Goto Y, Fukuma S, et al. Direct oral anticoagulants versus warfarin for preventing stroke and systemic embolic events among atrial fibrillation patients with chronic kidney disease (Review). Cochrane Database of Systematic Reviews. 2017;11.

25. Anne Sig Vestergaard, Flemming Skjoth, Torben Bjerregaard Larsen, et al. The importance of mean time in therapeutic range for complication rates in warfarin therapy of patients with atrial fibrillation. A systematic review and meta-regression analysis. 2017.

26. Deepalakshmi M, Christy Joseph, Carolyne Jacob, Arun KP, Ponnusankar S. Management of Warfarin Therapy: A New Point-Of-Care Monitoring Service by Community Pharmacists in India. J Young Pharm, 2018;10(3):350-353.

27. Laila Mahmoud Matalqah, Khaldoon Radaideh, Syed Azhar Syed Sulaiman1, Mohamed Azmi Hassali, Muhamad Ali, SK Abdul Kader. An instrument to measure anticoagulation knowledge among Malaysian community: A translation and validation study of the Oral Anticoagulation Knowledge (OAK) Test.

28. Sahimi Mohamed, Tariq Abdul Razak, Rosnani Hashim. Development of Knowledge of Anticoagulant Questionnaire: A Narrative Literature Review.

29. Chandresh B. Dumatar, Sandip S. Jadav, Aashutosh J. Patel, Utilization Pattern of Antiplatelet and Anticoagulant Medicines

Among the Patients Suffering From Atrial Fibrillation. Journal of Young Pharmacists, 2018; 10(1):82-85.

30. Amber L Briggs, Susan Bruce, et al. The development and performance validation of a tool to assess patient anticoagulation knowledge. Research in Social and Administrative Pharmacy. 2005; 1(1):40-59.

Patient's Knowledge Assessment on Vitamin K Antagonist